DR. BARBARA JUICING RECIPES FOR HIGH BLOOD PRESSURE

Unlock vitalty:Dr. Barbara's potent juicing remedies to tame high blood pressure. Transform your health with delicious recipes rooted in science and flavorful wellness solution

I0702676

Miguel Sofia

Table of Contents

COPYRIGHT © 2023

All rights reserved. No part of this publication may be reproduced, distributed, or transmitted in any form or by any means, including photocopying, recording, or other electronic or mechanical methods, without the prior written permission of the publisher, except in the case of brief quotations embodied in critical reviews and certain other noncommercial uses permitted by copyright law.

CHAPTER ONE

Introduction to Dr. Barbara's Approach to Herbal Juicing for High Blood Pressure

High blood pressure, or hypertension, is a common medical condition affecting millions worldwide. It's a significant risk factor for heart disease, stroke, and other cardiovascular complications. While medications are commonly prescribed to manage hypertension, many people seek alternative approaches to complement their treatment or to reduce reliance on pharmaceuticals. Dr. Barbara's approach to herbal juicing for high blood pressure offers a holistic and natural way to support cardiovascular health. In this comprehensive guide, we'll delve into the principles, benefits, and methods of Dr. Barbara's herbal juicing approach.

Understanding High Blood Pressure:

Before exploring Dr. Barbara's approach, it's crucial to understand what high blood pressure is and its implications on health. High blood pressure occurs when the force of blood against the artery walls is consistently too high. This condition puts strain on the heart and blood vessels, increasing the risk of serious health problems. Hypertension is often asymptomatic, earning it the nickname "the silent killer" as it can go undetected for years while causing damage to vital organs.

Conventional Treatment vs. Herbal Remedies:

Conventional treatment for high blood pressure typically involves prescription medications, lifestyle modifications, and dietary changes. While medications can effectively lower blood pressure, they may come with side effects and long-term dependency concerns. Herbal remedies offer an alternative or complementary approach that focuses on harnessing the therapeutic properties of plants to support cardiovascular health. Dr. Barbara's approach combines the wisdom of traditional herbalism with modern nutritional science to create potent and nourishing herbal juices.

Dr. Barbara's Philosophy and Approach:

Dr. Barbara's philosophy centers on the belief that nature provides abundant resources for healing and wellness. She advocates for a holistic approach that considers the interconnectedness of body, mind, and spirit in achieving optimal health. Her approach to herbal juicing for high blood pressure involves selecting specific herbs and fruits known for their cardiovascular benefits and blending them into delicious and nutritious juices. These juices are designed to not only lower blood pressure but also nourish the body with essential vitamins, minerals, and antioxidants.

Key Herbs and Ingredients:

Several herbs and ingredients are commonly featured in Dr. Barbara's herbal juices for high blood pressure. These include:

1. **Hawthorn Berry:** Known for its cardiovascular benefits, hawthorn berry is rich in flavonoids and antioxidants that help dilate blood vessels, improve blood flow, and regulate blood pressure.

2. **Beetroot:** Beetroot is a powerhouse of nutrients, including nitrates that convert into nitric oxide in the body, promoting vasodilation and lowering blood pressure.

3. **Garlic:** Garlic has long been valued for its medicinal properties, including its ability to lower blood pressure and improve circulation.

4. **Ginger:** Ginger possesses anti-inflammatory and vasodilatory properties, making it beneficial for cardiovascular health and blood pressure regulation.

5. **Celery:** Celery contains compounds called phthalides, which relax the muscles in the walls of the arteries, promoting blood flow and reducing blood pressure.

Benefits of Herbal Juicing for High Blood Pressure:

Herbal juicing offers several benefits for individuals with high blood pressure:

1. **Natural Approach:** Herbal juices provide a natural and holistic approach to managing high blood pressure, without the side effects associated with some medications.

2. **Nutritional Support:** Herbal juices are rich in essential nutrients, vitamins, and minerals that support overall cardiovascular health and well-being.

3. **Antioxidant Protection:** Many herbs and fruits used in herbal juicing are rich in antioxidants, which help protect against oxidative stress and inflammation associated with hypertension.

4. **Hydration:** Proper hydration is essential for maintaining healthy blood pressure levels, and herbal juices contribute to overall hydration while providing additional health benefits.

5. **Customization:** Dr. Barbara's approach allows for customization based on individual preferences and specific health needs, ensuring optimal results and compliance.

How to Incorporate Herbal Juicing into Your Routine:

Incorporating herbal juicing into your daily routine is simple and convenient:

1. **Choose Quality Ingredients:** Select fresh, organic herbs and fruits from reputable sources to ensure maximum potency and purity.

2. **Invest in a Juicer:** Purchase a high-quality juicer capable of extracting the maximum nutrients from your ingredients while minimizing oxidation.

3. **Experiment with Recipes:** Get creative with your herbal juice recipes, combining different herbs, fruits, and vegetables to suit your taste preferences and health goals.

4. **Drink Regularly:** Incorporate herbal juices into your daily routine, either as standalone beverages or as part of a balanced meal plan.

5. **Monitor Your Blood Pressure:** Regularly monitor your blood pressure levels and consult with a healthcare professional to assess the effectiveness of herbal juicing as part of your hypertension management strategy.

Conclusion:

Dr. Barbara's approach to herbal juicing for high blood pressure offers a natural, holistic, and effective way to support cardiovascular health. By harnessing the therapeutic properties of specific herbs and fruits, individuals can lower their blood pressure, improve circulation, and nourish their bodies with essential nutrients. With careful selection of ingredients, dedication to regular juicing, and consultation with healthcare professionals, herbal juicing can be a valuable addition to a comprehensive approach to managing hypertension and promoting overall well-being.

CHAPTER TWO

Understanding High Blood Pressure: Causes, Symptoms, and Risks

High blood pressure, also known as hypertension, is a prevalent medical condition characterized by elevated pressure within the arteries. It is a significant risk factor for cardiovascular diseases such as heart attack, stroke, and heart failure. Understanding the causes, symptoms, and risks associated with high blood pressure is crucial for effective prevention, management, and treatment of this condition.

Causes of High Blood Pressure:

High blood pressure can be classified into two main categories: primary (essential) hypertension and secondary hypertension.

1. **Primary Hypertension:** This form of hypertension develops gradually over time and has no identifiable cause. It is thought to be the result of a combination of genetic, lifestyle, and environmental factors. Risk factors for primary hypertension include obesity, unhealthy diet, lack of physical activity, stress, and aging.

2. **Secondary Hypertension:** Secondary hypertension is caused by an underlying medical condition or medication. Common causes include kidney disease, adrenal gland disorders, thyroid disorders, obstructive sleep apnea, certain

medications (such as oral contraceptives, decongestants, and nonsteroidal anti-inflammatory drugs), and illegal drugs (such as cocaine and amphetamines).

Symptoms of High Blood Pressure:

High blood pressure is often asymptomatic, meaning it does not typically cause noticeable symptoms until it reaches a severe or life-threatening level. This is why hypertension is often referred to as "the silent killer." However, some people may experience symptoms such as:

1. **Headaches:** Severe headaches, especially in the back of the head, can be a symptom of high blood pressure.

2. **Dizziness or Lightheadedness:** Feeling dizzy or lightheaded, particularly when standing up quickly, can occur with high blood pressure.

3. **Blurred or Double Vision:** Vision changes, including blurred or double vision, may occur in individuals with severely elevated blood pressure.

4. **Chest Pain:** Chest pain, especially during physical activity or exertion, can be a symptom of high blood pressure-related heart problems.

5. **Shortness of Breath:** Difficulty breathing or shortness of breath may occur in individuals with high blood pressure-related heart failure or pulmonary edema.

It's important to note that these symptoms can also be indicative of other medical conditions, and not everyone with high blood pressure will experience them.

Risks Associated with High Blood Pressure:

Untreated or poorly controlled high blood pressure can lead to serious health complications and increase the risk of:

1. **Heart Disease:** High blood pressure can damage the arteries and heart muscle, increasing the risk of coronary artery disease, heart attack, and heart failure.

2. **Stroke:** Hypertension is a leading cause of stroke, which occurs when blood flow to the brain is disrupted due to a blockage or rupture of a blood vessel.

3. **Kidney Damage:** High blood pressure can damage the blood vessels in the kidneys, leading to kidney disease or kidney failure.

4. **Vision Loss:** Hypertension can damage the blood vessels in the eyes, increasing the risk of vision problems and even blindness.

5. **Peripheral Artery Disease:** High blood pressure can cause narrowing and hardening of the arteries in the legs and arms, leading to decreased blood flow and increased risk of complications such as leg pain and tissue damage.

6. **Aneurysm:** Chronic high blood pressure can weaken the walls of blood vessels, increasing the risk of aneurysm formation, particularly in the aorta (the body's main artery).

Conclusion:

High blood pressure is a common and serious medical condition that can have devastating consequences if left untreated. Understanding the causes, symptoms, and risks associated with hypertension is essential for early detection, prevention, and management. Lifestyle modifications, including a healthy diet, regular exercise, stress management, and medication when necessary, play a crucial role in controlling blood pressure and reducing the risk of complications. Regular monitoring of blood pressure and routine medical check-ups are important for individuals at risk of or diagnosed with hypertension.

CHAPTER THREE

The Role of Nutrition in Managing High Blood Pressure

Nutrition plays a crucial role in managing high blood pressure (hypertension). A healthy diet can help control blood pressure levels, reduce the risk of cardiovascular complications, and improve overall health and well-being. In this comprehensive guide, we'll explore the impact of nutrition on hypertension management, including dietary recommendations, nutrient considerations, and lifestyle modifications.

Dietary Recommendations for Hypertension Management:

1. **DASH Diet:** The Dietary Approaches to Stop Hypertension (DASH) diet is a well-researched dietary pattern specifically designed to lower blood pressure. It emphasizes fruits, vegetables, whole grains, lean proteins, and low-fat dairy products while limiting sodium, saturated fats, and added sugars.

2. **High-Potassium Foods:** Potassium helps regulate blood pressure by counteracting the effects of sodium and relaxing blood vessel walls. Foods rich in potassium include bananas, oranges, spinach, sweet potatoes, and avocado.

3. **Magnesium-Rich Foods:** Magnesium plays a role in blood pressure regulation and muscle function. Magnesium-rich

foods include nuts, seeds, whole grains, leafy greens, and legumes.

4. **Calcium-Rich Foods:** Calcium is important for maintaining healthy blood pressure levels and bone health. Good sources of calcium include dairy products, fortified plant-based milks, leafy greens, and tofu.

5. **Omega-3 Fatty Acids:** Omega-3 fatty acids found in fatty fish (such as salmon, mackerel, and sardines), flaxseeds, chia seeds, and walnuts have been associated with lower blood pressure and reduced risk of heart disease.

6. **Fiber-Rich Foods:** Fiber helps lower blood pressure by promoting satiety, improving digestive health, and reducing cholesterol levels. Fiber-rich foods include whole grains, fruits, vegetables, legumes, and nuts.

Nutrient Considerations for Hypertension Management:

1. **Sodium Reduction:** High sodium intake is strongly linked to elevated blood pressure. Limiting sodium consumption by avoiding processed foods, using herbs and spices for flavoring instead of salt, and choosing low-sodium alternatives can help control blood pressure.

2. **Moderate Alcohol Consumption:** Excessive alcohol consumption can raise blood pressure and increase the risk

of cardiovascular disease. Limiting alcohol intake to moderate levels (up to one drink per day for women and up to two drinks per day for men) is recommended.

3. **Limit Saturated and Trans Fats:** Saturated and trans fats can raise cholesterol levels and contribute to hypertension and heart disease. Limiting intake of foods high in these fats, such as fatty meats, full-fat dairy products, and processed foods, is beneficial for blood pressure management.

4. **Monitor Caffeine Intake:** While moderate caffeine consumption is generally considered safe for most individuals, excessive caffeine intake can temporarily raise blood pressure. Individuals sensitive to caffeine should monitor their intake from coffee, tea, energy drinks, and other sources.

5. **Hydration:** Adequate hydration is important for maintaining healthy blood pressure levels. Drinking plenty of water and consuming hydrating foods such as fruits and vegetables can help prevent dehydration, which can contribute to elevated blood pressure.

Lifestyle Modifications for Hypertension Management:

In addition to dietary changes, certain lifestyle modifications can further support hypertension management:

1. **Regular Exercise:** Engaging in regular physical activity, such as brisk walking, swimming, cycling, or strength training, can help lower blood pressure, improve cardiovascular health, and manage weight.

2. **Stress Management:** Chronic stress can contribute to elevated blood pressure. Practicing relaxation techniques such as deep breathing, meditation, yoga, and mindfulness can help reduce stress levels and promote overall well-being.

3. **Weight Management:** Maintaining a healthy weight through a balanced diet and regular exercise is essential for blood pressure control. Losing excess weight, particularly abdominal fat, can significantly lower blood pressure levels.

4. **Smoking Cessation:** Smoking and exposure to secondhand smoke can raise blood pressure and increase the risk of heart disease and stroke. Quitting smoking and avoiding exposure to tobacco smoke are crucial for hypertension management.

Conclusion:

Nutrition plays a central role in managing high blood pressure. Following a healthy diet rich in fruits, vegetables, whole grains, lean proteins, and healthy fats while limiting sodium, saturated fats, and added sugars can help control blood pressure levels and reduce the risk of cardiovascular complications. In addition to dietary changes, lifestyle modifications such as regular exercise, stress management, weight management, and smoking cessation are important components of a comprehensive approach to hypertension management. Consulting with a healthcare professional or registered dietitian can provide personalized guidance and support for individuals seeking to manage their blood pressure through nutrition and lifestyle modifications.

CHAPTER FOUR

Dr. Barbara's Principles of Herbal Healing and Blood Pressure Regulation

Dr. Barbara's approach to herbal healing and blood pressure regulation is rooted in the principles of holistic health and traditional herbalism. With a deep understanding of botanical medicine and a commitment to natural healing, Dr. Barbara has developed a comprehensive approach to supporting cardiovascular health and managing high blood pressure. In this guide, we'll explore Dr. Barbara's principles, methods, and key herbs for herbal healing and blood pressure regulation.

Holistic Approach to Healing:

Dr. Barbara embraces a holistic approach to healing, recognizing the interconnectedness of the body, mind, and spirit in achieving optimal health and well-being. Rather than treating symptoms in isolation, she addresses the underlying root causes of health imbalances, considering the individual as a whole. This holistic perspective acknowledges the importance of nutrition, lifestyle factors, emotional well-being, and environmental influences in supporting overall health and vitality.

Power of Botanical Medicine:

Central to Dr. Barbara's approach is the power of botanical medicine in promoting health and healing. She draws upon the rich tradition of herbalism, which has been used for centuries by cultures around the world to treat various ailments and support wellness. Herbs are valued not only for their therapeutic properties but also for their gentle and synergistic effects on the body, offering a natural and holistic alternative to conventional medications.

Blood Pressure Regulation with Herbs:

Dr. Barbara recognizes the potential of specific herbs to regulate blood pressure and support cardiovascular health. By selecting herbs with vasodilatory, hypotensive, and cardioprotective properties, she creates herbal formulations and blends aimed at lowering blood pressure, improving circulation, and strengthening the heart and blood vessels. These herbs work synergistically to address the underlying factors contributing to hypertension while nourishing the body with essential nutrients and antioxidants.

Key Herbs for Blood Pressure Regulation:

1. **Hawthorn Berry (Crataegus spp.):** Hawthorn berry is a cornerstone herb in Dr. Barbara's approach to blood pressure regulation. Rich in flavonoids and antioxidants, hawthorn berry helps dilate blood vessels, improve blood flow, and strengthen the heart muscle. It is also known for its calming and stress-reducing effects, which can benefit individuals with hypertension.

2. **Garlic (Allium sativum):** Garlic has been used for centuries for its medicinal properties, including its ability to lower blood pressure and cholesterol levels. It contains sulfur compounds that promote vasodilation and inhibit the production of angiotensin II, a hormone that raises blood pressure.

3. **Hibiscus (Hibiscus sabdariffa):** Hibiscus tea is a popular herbal remedy for hypertension due to its diuretic and antihypertensive properties. It contains anthocyanins and polyphenols that help relax blood vessels, reduce inflammation, and lower blood pressure levels.

4. **Olive Leaf (Olea europaea):** Olive leaf extract is rich in oleuropein, a compound with antioxidant and anti-inflammatory properties. It helps relax blood vessels, improve circulation, and reduce blood pressure levels by inhibiting the enzyme responsible for constricting blood vessels.

5. **Celery Seed (Apium graveolens):** Celery seed is traditionally used as a diuretic and antihypertensive herb. It contains compounds called phthalides, which help relax the muscles in the walls of blood vessels, leading to lower blood pressure levels.

Methods of Herbal Administration:

Dr. Barbara employs various methods of herbal administration to deliver the therapeutic benefits of herbs effectively. These may include:

1. **Herbal Teas:** Herbal teas are a convenient and soothing way to consume medicinal herbs. Dr. Barbara often recommends brewing herbal teas using dried herbs or tea bags for easy preparation and consumption.

2. **Tinctures:** Tinctures are liquid herbal extracts made by soaking herbs in alcohol or glycerin to extract their active constituents. They are highly concentrated and can be easily dosed, making them a convenient option for blood pressure regulation.

3. **Herbal Capsules or Tablets:** For individuals who prefer a more convenient and portable option, herbal capsules or tablets containing standardized herbal extracts may be recommended by Dr. Barbara. These provide a consistent dosage of herbs and can be taken with water or food.

4. **Herbal Juices:** Herbal juices offer a refreshing and nourishing way to consume medicinal herbs. By blending fresh herbs with fruits and vegetables, Dr. Barbara creates delicious and nutrient-rich juices that support cardiovascular health and blood pressure regulation.

Conclusion:

Dr. Barbara's principles of herbal healing and blood pressure regulation emphasize a holistic approach to health, the power of botanical medicine, and the therapeutic benefits of specific herbs in supporting cardiovascular wellness. By incorporating key herbs known for their blood pressure-lowering properties into various herbal formulations and blends, Dr. Barbara provides natural and effective solutions for individuals seeking to manage hypertension and promote overall well-being. With a focus on personalized care and patient empowerment, Dr. Barbara's approach empowers individuals to take control of their health and embrace the healing potential of nature's pharmacy.

CHAPTER FIVE

The Benefits of Herbal Juicing for Lowering Blood Pressure

Herbal juicing offers a natural and effective approach to lowering blood pressure and promoting cardiovascular health. By combining specific herbs with fruits and vegetables, herbal juices deliver potent doses of therapeutic compounds that support healthy blood pressure levels and overall well-being. In this guide, we'll explore the benefits of herbal juicing for lowering blood pressure and how it can complement conventional treatments and lifestyle modifications.

1. Rich in Cardiovascular-Protective Nutrients:

Herbal juices are packed with vitamins, minerals, antioxidants, and phytonutrients that support cardiovascular health. Fruits and vegetables such as berries, leafy greens, citrus fruits, and beets are particularly rich in potassium, magnesium, vitamin C, and dietary nitrates, which have been shown to help lower blood pressure and improve heart health.

2. Natural Vasodilators and Antihypertensive Compounds:

Many herbs used in herbal juicing possess vasodilatory and antihypertensive properties, meaning they help relax blood vessels and lower blood pressure. Herbs like hawthorn berry, garlic, ginger, celery seed, and olive leaf contain compounds that promote vasodilation, improve blood flow, and reduce the resistance of blood vessels, resulting in lower blood pressure readings.

3. Supports Healthy Circulation:

Herbal juices support healthy circulation by improving blood flow throughout the body. Ingredients like ginger, turmeric, cayenne pepper, and hibiscus help dilate blood vessels, prevent blood clots, and reduce inflammation, promoting optimal circulation and oxygen delivery to tissues and organs.

4. Reduces Oxidative Stress and Inflammation:

Chronic oxidative stress and inflammation are key contributors to hypertension and cardiovascular disease. The antioxidants found in herbs and fruits used in herbal juicing, such as berries, turmeric, ginger, and green tea, help neutralize free radicals, reduce inflammation, and protect against oxidative damage to blood vessels, thus lowering blood pressure and reducing the risk of heart disease.

5. Supports Weight Management:

Maintaining a healthy weight is essential for blood pressure control. Herbal juices, when incorporated into a balanced diet and lifestyle, can support weight management efforts by providing low-calorie, nutrient-dense options that promote satiety, hydration, and overall well-being. Additionally, certain herbs like ginger and cayenne pepper have thermogenic properties that may boost metabolism and aid in weight loss.

6. Hydration and Electrolyte Balance:

Proper hydration and electrolyte balance are crucial for maintaining healthy blood pressure levels. Herbal juices contribute to hydration while providing essential electrolytes like potassium and magnesium, which help regulate fluid balance, muscle function, and blood pressure. Hydrating with herbal juices can prevent dehydration, a common cause of elevated blood pressure.

7. Promotes Detoxification and Kidney Health:

The kidneys play a vital role in regulating blood pressure by balancing fluid and electrolyte levels in the body. Herbal juices containing diuretic herbs like dandelion, parsley, and cilantro can support kidney function and promote detoxification, helping to remove excess sodium and fluid from the body and lower blood pressure.

Conclusion:

Herbal juicing offers numerous benefits for lowering blood pressure and supporting cardiovascular health. By harnessing the therapeutic properties of herbs and combining them with nutrient-rich fruits and vegetables, herbal juices provide a natural and delicious way to promote healthy blood pressure levels, reduce the risk of heart disease, and enhance overall well-being. Incorporating herbal juices into a balanced diet and lifestyle can complement conventional treatments and lifestyle modifications for hypertension, offering a holistic approach to cardiovascular wellness. As with any dietary regimen, it's essential to consult with a healthcare professional or registered dietitian to ensure that herbal juicing is safe and appropriate for individual health needs and goals.

CHAPTER SIX

Preparing Your Body for the Herbal Juicing Protocol: Tips and Guidelines

Embarking on an herbal juicing protocol for managing high blood pressure requires some preparation to ensure success and maximize benefits. By taking proactive steps to prepare your body, mind, and kitchen, you can set yourself up for a smooth and effective juicing experience. Here are some tips and guidelines to help you prepare for your herbal juicing journey:

1. Consult with a Healthcare Professional: Before starting any new dietary regimen or herbal protocol, it's essential to consult with a healthcare professional, especially if you have underlying health conditions or are taking medications. Your healthcare provider can offer personalized guidance and ensure that herbal juicing is safe and appropriate for your individual needs.

2. Set Clear Goals and Expectations: Define your goals for herbal juicing, whether it's lowering blood pressure, improving overall health, increasing energy levels, or detoxifying the body. Setting clear and realistic goals will help you stay motivated and track your progress throughout the juicing protocol.

3. Gradually Transition to a Plant-Based Diet: If you're not already following a plant-based diet, consider gradually transitioning to one in the days or weeks leading up to your herbal juicing protocol. Incorporate more fruits, vegetables, whole grains, and plant-based proteins into your meals to prepare your body for the nutrient-rich juices it will be receiving.

4. Hydrate Well: Proper hydration is essential for supporting detoxification, digestion, and overall health. Start increasing your water intake in the days leading up to your juicing protocol to ensure that your body is well-hydrated and prepared for the increased fluid intake from herbal juices.

5. Stock Up on Fresh Ingredients: Gather a variety of fresh fruits, vegetables, and herbs for your juicing protocol. Choose organic produce whenever possible to minimize exposure to pesticides and maximize nutrient content. Wash and prepare your ingredients ahead of time to streamline the juicing process.

6. Invest in a High-Quality Juicer: Invest in a high-quality juicer capable of extracting the maximum nutrients from your ingredients while minimizing oxidation. Choose a juicer that meets your needs and budget, whether it's a centrifugal juicer, masticating juicer, or cold-press juicer.

7. Gather Essential Kitchen Tools: In addition to a juicer, gather essential kitchen tools and accessories for juicing, such as cutting boards, sharp knives, measuring cups, and storage containers for fresh juice. Having everything you need within reach will make the juicing process more efficient and enjoyable.

8. Plan Your Juicing Schedule: Create a juicing schedule that works for your lifestyle and preferences. Decide whether you'll be juicing once a day, multiple times a day, or on specific days of the week. Set aside time in your schedule for juicing, and consider prepping larger batches of juice to save time.

9. Practice Mindful Eating: In the days leading up to your juicing protocol, practice mindful eating by paying attention to hunger cues, savoring each bite, and chewing your food thoroughly. Mindful eating can help you develop a deeper connection with your body and cultivate healthier eating habits.

10. Stay Positive and Open-Minded: Approach your herbal juicing protocol with a positive mindset and an open heart. Embrace the opportunity for nourishment, healing, and transformation, and trust in the wisdom of nature to support your journey to better health and well-being.

By following these tips and guidelines, you can prepare your body, mind, and kitchen for a successful herbal juicing protocol. Remember to listen to your body, honor your individual needs, and enjoy the journey to vibrant health and vitality with each delicious sip of herbal juice.

CHAPTER SEVEN

Selecting the right herbs

Selecting the right herbs for juicing to lower blood pressure requires careful consideration of their therapeutic properties, safety profile, and potential synergistic effects. By choosing herbs known for their vasodilatory, hypotensive, and cardioprotective properties, you can create delicious and effective herbal juices that support cardiovascular health and promote healthy blood pressure levels. Here are some key herbs to consider for juicing to lower blood pressure:

1. Hawthorn Berry (Crataegus spp.): Hawthorn berry is a potent herb known for its cardiovascular benefits, including its ability to dilate blood vessels, improve blood flow, and strengthen the heart muscle. It contains flavonoids and antioxidants that help lower blood pressure and reduce the risk of heart disease. Include fresh or dried hawthorn berries in your herbal juices to support overall cardiovascular health.

2. Garlic (Allium sativum): Garlic is a culinary herb with powerful medicinal properties, including its ability to lower blood pressure and improve circulation. It contains sulfur compounds that promote vasodilation, reduce cholesterol levels, and prevent blood clot formation. Add fresh garlic cloves to your herbal juices for a flavorful and heart-healthy boost.

3. Beetroot (Beta vulgaris): Beetroot is rich in dietary nitrates, which convert into nitric oxide in the body, promoting vasodilation and improving blood flow. Drinking beetroot juice has been shown to lower blood pressure and enhance exercise performance. Incorporate fresh beetroot into your herbal juices for a vibrant color and cardiovascular support.

4. Ginger (Zingiber officinale): Ginger is a versatile herb with anti-inflammatory and vasodilatory properties that support cardiovascular health. It helps relax blood vessels, improve circulation, and lower blood pressure. Fresh ginger root adds a zesty flavor and therapeutic benefits to your herbal juices.

5. Celery (Apium graveolens): Celery contains compounds called phthalides, which help relax the muscles in the walls of blood vessels, leading to lower blood pressure levels. Including fresh celery stalks or leaves in your herbal juices adds a refreshing and hydrating element while supporting cardiovascular health.

6. Turmeric (Curcuma longa): Turmeric is a potent anti-inflammatory herb with cardiovascular benefits, including its ability to lower blood pressure, improve endothelial function, and reduce oxidative stress. Add fresh turmeric root or powdered turmeric to your herbal juices for its vibrant color and therapeutic effects.

7. Hibiscus (Hibiscus sabdariffa): Hibiscus tea is a popular herbal remedy for hypertension due to its diuretic and antihypertensive properties. It contains anthocyanins and polyphenols that help relax blood vessels, reduce inflammation, and lower blood pressure levels. Brew hibiscus tea and use it as a base for your herbal juices or add dried hibiscus flowers to your juice blends.

8. Parsley (Petroselinum crispum): Parsley is a nutrient-rich herb that supports cardiovascular health and kidney function. It contains compounds like flavonoids and vitamins C and K, which help regulate blood pressure and promote fluid balance. Include fresh parsley leaves in your herbal juices for their detoxifying and heart-healthy benefits.

9. Lemon (Citrus limon): Lemon is a citrus fruit rich in vitamin C and antioxidants that support cardiovascular health. It helps improve blood circulation, reduce inflammation, and lower blood pressure levels. Squeeze fresh lemon juice into your herbal juices for a tangy flavor and additional health benefits.

10. Cinnamon (Cinnamomum verum): Cinnamon is a warming spice with cardiovascular benefits, including its ability to improve blood circulation, lower cholesterol levels, and regulate blood sugar. Add powdered cinnamon to your herbal juices for its delicious flavor and heart-healthy effects.

When selecting herbs for juicing to lower blood pressure, choose organic, high-quality ingredients from reputable sources whenever possible. Experiment with different combinations of herbs, fruits, and vegetables to create flavorful and therapeutic juice blends that support cardiovascular health and promote optimal blood pressure levels. Remember to consult with a healthcare professional or registered dietitian before starting any new herbal regimen, especially if you have underlying health conditions or are taking medications.

CHAPTER EIGHT

Dr. Barbara's recommended juice recipes for high blood pressure

Dr. Barbara's recommended juice recipes for high blood pressure are carefully crafted to combine specific herbs, fruits, and vegetables known for their cardiovascular benefits and blood pressure-lowering properties. These delicious and nourishing juice blends provide a natural and effective way to support cardiovascular health and promote optimal blood pressure levels. Here are some of Dr. Barbara's favorite juice recipes for high blood pressure:

1. Heart Health Booster:

- 1 cup fresh spinach leaves
- 1/2 cup fresh kale leaves
- 1/2 cucumber
- 1 green apple
- 1/2 lemon (peeled)
- 1-inch piece of fresh ginger root
- Handful of parsley

2. Blood Pressure Balancer:

- 1 beetroot (medium-sized, peeled)

- 2 carrots

- 1 celery stalk

- 1/2 cucumber

- Handful of fresh cilantro

- 1/2 lemon (peeled)

- 1-inch piece of fresh turmeric root

3. Cardiovascular Support Blend:

- 1 cup mixed berries (such as strawberries, blueberries, and raspberries)

- 1/2 cup fresh spinach leaves

- 1/2 cup fresh kale leaves

- 1/2 cucumber

- 1 green apple

- 1/2 lemon (peeled)

- Handful of fresh mint leaves

4. Hibiscus Berry Refresher:

- 2 tablespoons dried hibiscus flowers

- 1 cup mixed berries (such as strawberries, raspberries, and blackberries)

- 1/2 cucumber

- 1/2 lemon (peeled)

- 1-inch piece of fresh ginger root

- Handful of fresh mint leaves

5. Ginger Beet Cleanse:

- 1 beetroot (medium-sized, peeled)

- 1 apple (green or red)

- 1/2 cucumber

- 1-inch piece of fresh ginger root

- 1/2 lemon (peeled)

- Handful of fresh parsley

6. Green Goddess Detoxifier:

- 2 cups fresh spinach leaves

- 1/2 cucumber

- 1 green apple

- 1/2 lemon (peeled)

- Handful of fresh cilantro

- Handful of fresh mint leaves

7. Citrus Sunshine Elixir:

- 2 oranges (peeled)

- 1/2 grapefruit (peeled)

- 1/2 lemon (peeled)

- 1-inch piece of fresh ginger root

- Handful of fresh basil leaves

8. Turmeric Tonic Delight:

- 1-inch piece of fresh turmeric root

- 1 apple (green or red)

- 1/2 cucumber

- 1/2 lemon (peeled)

- Handful of fresh parsley

- Pinch of black pepper (to enhance turmeric absorption)

9. Garlic Greens Powerhouse:

- 2 cloves of garlic

- 1 cup fresh spinach leaves

- 1/2 cucumber

- 1 green apple

- 1/2 lemon (peeled)

- Handful of fresh cilantro

- Handful of fresh parsley

10. Berry Blast Antioxidant Booster:

- 1 cup mixed berries (such as blueberries, strawberries, and raspberries)

- 1/2 cucumber

- 1/2 lemon (peeled)

- Handful of fresh basil leaves

- Handful of fresh mint leaves

Instructions:

1. Wash all fruits, vegetables, and herbs thoroughly.

2. Peel and chop ingredients as needed to fit into your juicer.

3. Juice all ingredients using a high-quality juicer.

4. Stir the juice well and pour into a glass.

5. Enjoy immediately for maximum freshness and nutrient benefits.

These juice recipes are designed to be delicious, refreshing, and packed with nutrients that support cardiovascular health and help lower blood pressure naturally. Incorporate them into your daily routine as part of a balanced diet and lifestyle for optimal results. Remember to consult with a healthcare professional or registered dietitian before starting any new dietary regimen, especially if you have underlying health conditions or are taking medications.

CHAPTER NINE

Incorporating herbal supplements

Incorporating herbal supplements can be a valuable addition to your blood pressure management regimen, offering natural alternatives to conventional medications and complementing lifestyle modifications. When selecting herbal supplements for blood pressure support, it's essential to choose high-quality products from reputable sources and consult with a healthcare professional or qualified herbalist to ensure safety and effectiveness. Here are some herbal supplements commonly used to support blood pressure management:

1. Hawthorn (Crataegus spp.): Hawthorn is a well-known herb for cardiovascular health, with research supporting its use in lowering blood pressure and improving heart function. Hawthorn extracts or capsules are commonly used to support overall cardiovascular health and may help regulate blood pressure levels over time.

2. Garlic (Allium sativum): Garlic has been traditionally used for its cardiovascular benefits, including its ability to lower blood pressure and improve circulation. Garlic supplements, such as aged garlic extract, can provide the benefits of garlic without the odor or digestive issues associated with raw garlic consumption.

3. Olive Leaf (Olea europaea): Olive leaf extract contains compounds that have been shown to lower blood pressure and improve endothelial function. It may help relax blood vessels, reduce inflammation, and protect against oxidative stress. Olive leaf supplements are available in capsule or liquid form.

4. Fish Oil (Omega-3 Fatty Acids): Fish oil supplements are rich in omega-3 fatty acids, which have been shown to have cardiovascular benefits, including lowering blood pressure, reducing triglyceride levels, and improving heart health. Choose high-quality fish oil supplements sourced from wild-caught, cold-water fish for optimal potency and purity.

5. Beetroot Extract: Beetroot contains dietary nitrates that convert into nitric oxide in the body, promoting vasodilation and improving blood flow. Beetroot supplements or beetroot powder can help lower blood pressure and enhance exercise performance. Look for standardized beetroot extracts for consistency and potency.

6. Magnesium: Magnesium is an essential mineral that plays a crucial role in regulating blood pressure and cardiovascular function. Magnesium supplements may help lower blood pressure in individuals with magnesium deficiency or insufficiency. Choose magnesium supplements in forms such as magnesium citrate or magnesium glycinate for better absorption.

7. Hibiscus (Hibiscus sabdariffa): Hibiscus tea has been studied for its potential to lower blood pressure due to its diuretic and antihypertensive properties. Hibiscus supplements, such as dried hibiscus flower extracts or capsules, can provide a convenient way to incorporate this herb into your blood pressure management regimen.

8. Cinnamon (Cinnamomum verum): Cinnamon has been shown to have antihypertensive effects and may help lower blood pressure by improving insulin sensitivity and reducing inflammation. Cinnamon supplements or cinnamon extract capsules can be used to supplement dietary intake and support blood pressure management.

9. Celery Seed Extract: Celery seed extract contains compounds that have been studied for their potential to lower blood pressure by promoting vasodilation and diuresis. Celery seed supplements may help support cardiovascular health and complement dietary and lifestyle interventions for blood pressure management.

10. Coenzyme Q10 (CoQ10): Coenzyme Q10 is a powerful antioxidant that supports heart health and cellular energy production. CoQ10 supplements have been shown to help lower blood pressure and improve cardiovascular function, especially in individuals with CoQ10 deficiency or certain medical conditions.

Before incorporating herbal supplements into your blood pressure management regimen, it's essential to consult with a healthcare professional or qualified herbalist to ensure safety and efficacy, especially if you have underlying health conditions or are taking medications. They can provide personalized recommendations based on your individual needs and help you navigate the world of herbal medicine effectively. Additionally, monitor your blood pressure regularly and communicate any changes or concerns with your healthcare provider for optimal management and support.

CHAPTER TEN

Long-term lifestyle strategies

Long-term lifestyle strategies play a crucial role in maintaining healthy blood pressure levels through herbal juicing and nutrition. By incorporating sustainable dietary habits, herbal remedies, and lifestyle modifications into your daily routine, you can support cardiovascular health, reduce the risk of hypertension-related complications, and promote overall well-being. Here are some long-term lifestyle strategies for maintaining healthy blood pressure levels through herbal juicing and nutrition:

1. Adopt a Balanced and Nutrient-Rich Diet: Focus on consuming a balanced diet rich in fruits, vegetables, whole grains, lean proteins, and healthy fats. Incorporate a variety of colorful fruits and vegetables into your meals to ensure a diverse intake of vitamins, minerals, antioxidants, and phytonutrients that support cardiovascular health.

2. Embrace Herbal Juicing as a Regular Practice: Make herbal juicing a regular part of your daily or weekly routine to support blood pressure management and overall health. Experiment with different combinations of herbs, fruits, and vegetables to create delicious and nutritious juice blends that promote optimal blood pressure levels and provide essential nutrients.

3. Prioritize Potassium-Rich Foods: Include potassium-rich foods in your diet, such as bananas, oranges, spinach, sweet potatoes, avocado, and tomatoes. Potassium helps regulate blood pressure by counteracting the effects of sodium and promoting vasodilation, making it an essential nutrient for cardiovascular health.

4. Limit Sodium Intake: Reduce your intake of processed foods, fast food, and high-sodium snacks, which can contribute to elevated blood pressure levels. Opt for fresh, whole foods and use herbs, spices, and natural flavorings to enhance the taste of your meals without relying on excess salt.

5. Incorporate Heart-Healthy Fats: Include sources of heart-healthy fats in your diet, such as oily fish (salmon, mackerel, sardines), nuts, seeds, olive oil, and avocado. These fats provide essential omega-3 fatty acids, which support cardiovascular health and may help lower blood pressure.

6. Stay Hydrated: Drink plenty of water throughout the day to stay hydrated and support optimal blood pressure levels. Herbal teas, infused water, and hydrating herbal juices can also contribute to your daily fluid intake and provide additional health benefits.

7. Maintain a Healthy Weight: Maintain a healthy weight through a combination of balanced nutrition, regular physical activity, and lifestyle modifications. Aim for a body mass index (BMI) within the healthy range and prioritize gradual, sustainable weight loss if necessary to support blood pressure management.

8. Engage in Regular Physical Activity: Incorporate regular exercise into your routine to support cardiovascular health, improve circulation, and lower blood pressure. Aim for at least 150 minutes of moderate-intensity aerobic activity or 75 minutes of vigorous-intensity aerobic activity per week, along with muscle-strengthening exercises on two or more days per week.

9. Manage Stress Effectively: Practice stress-reduction techniques such as deep breathing, meditation, yoga, mindfulness, and progressive muscle relaxation to manage stress levels and promote relaxation. Chronic stress can contribute to elevated blood pressure, so prioritizing stress management is essential for long-term cardiovascular health.

10. Get Quality Sleep: Prioritize quality sleep by maintaining a consistent sleep schedule, creating a relaxing bedtime routine, and optimizing your sleep environment. Aim for 7-9 hours of restful sleep per night to support overall health and blood pressure regulation.

11. Monitor Your Blood Pressure Regularly: Keep track of your blood pressure readings regularly, either at home or with the guidance of a healthcare professional. Monitoring your blood pressure allows you to track changes over time, identify patterns, and make necessary adjustments to your lifestyle and treatment plan.

By incorporating these long-term lifestyle strategies into your daily routine, you can maintain healthy blood pressure levels, support cardiovascular health, and promote overall well-being through herbal juicing and nutrition. Remember to consult with a healthcare professional or registered dietitian for personalized guidance and recommendations based on your individual health needs and goals.

BONUS: SOME HERBAL REMEDIES TO KNOW

Goldenseal:

Definition: Goldenseal, scientifically known as Hydrastis canadensis, is a perennial herb native to North America. It has a long history of use in traditional Native American medicine and later in folk medicine for its potential health benefits.

Ingredients: Goldenseal root contains various bioactive compounds, including alkaloids (such as berberine and hydrastine), flavonoids, and volatile oils. These compounds are believed to contribute to the herb's medicinal properties, including its potential as an antimicrobial, anti-inflammatory, and immune enhancer.

How to Prepare: Goldenseal is typically consumed as an herbal tea, tincture, or in supplement form (such as capsules or tablets). To make tea, dried goldenseal root or leaves are steeped in hot water for several minutes before being strained and consumed.

Dosage: The appropriate dosage of goldenseal can vary depending on factors such as age, health status, and the specific preparation being used. It's important to follow the recommended dosage on the product label or consult with a qualified herbalist or healthcare professional for personalized guidance.

How to Use: Goldenseal tea, tincture, or supplements are typically taken orally. It's often used to support immune function, promote digestive health, and soothe inflammation.

Side Effects: Goldenseal is generally considered safe for most people when used in moderate amounts. However, some individuals may experience mild side effects such as gastrointestinal upset or allergic reactions. It may also interact with certain medications or have adverse effects in individuals with certain health conditions, such as high blood pressure or pregnancy. It's important to use goldenseal under the guidance of a healthcare professional and to discontinue use if any adverse effects occur.

Bio Ferro Tonic:

Definition: Bio Ferro Tonic is a dietary supplement primarily composed of herbs and minerals. It's often marketed as a natural way to support overall health, particularly by promoting blood health and circulation.

Ingredients: Typical ingredients in Bio Ferro Tonic may include a blend of herbs such as burdock root, yellow dock root, sarsaparilla root, and cascara sagrada bark, along with minerals like iron and potassium phosphate.

How to Prepare: Bio Ferro Tonic usually comes in liquid form and is typically taken orally. It's important to follow the instructions on the product label for dosage and administration.

Dosage: The dosage can vary depending on the specific product and individual needs. It's crucial to consult with a healthcare professional or follow the recommended dosage on the product label to avoid potential side effects.

How to Use: Bio Ferro Tonic is often taken by adding the recommended dosage to water or juice and consuming it orally. It's important to shake the bottle well before use and store it according to the manufacturer's instructions.

Side Effects: While Bio Ferro Tonic is generally considered safe when used as directed, some individuals may experience side effects such as digestive discomfort, allergic reactions, or interactions with medications. It's essential to consult with a healthcare provider before starting any new supplement regimen, especially if you have underlying health conditions or are taking medications.

Bladderwrack:

Definition: Bladderwrack is a type of seaweed or marine algae commonly used in traditional medicine and as a dietary supplement. It's known for its potential health benefits, particularly related to thyroid health and weight management.

Ingredients: Bladderwrack contains various nutrients, including iodine, vitamins, minerals, and antioxidants. The primary active components are iodine and fucoidan, a type of carbohydrate found in brown seaweeds.

How to Prepare: Bladderwrack supplements are available in various forms, including capsules, powders, and liquid extracts. They can be taken orally with water or added to smoothies and other beverages.

Dosage: The appropriate dosage of bladderwrack can vary based on factors such as age, health status, and the specific product being used. It's essential to follow the recommended dosage on the product label or consult with a healthcare professional for personalized guidance.

How to Use: Bladderwrack supplements are typically taken orally, either with water or mixed into food or beverages. It's important to follow the instructions on the product label and avoid exceeding the recommended dosage.

Side Effects: While bladderwrack is generally considered safe for most people when used in moderation, excessive intake of iodine from bladderwrack supplements can cause thyroid dysfunction and other adverse effects. Individuals with thyroid disorders, iodine sensitivity, or certain medical conditions should exercise caution and consult with a healthcare provider before using bladderwrack supplements. Common side effects may include digestive upset, allergic reactions, or interactions with medications.

Blood Purifier:

Definition: Blood purifiers are herbal remedies or dietary supplements believed to cleanse or detoxify the blood, often promoting overall health and well-being. They are thought to support the body's natural detoxification processes and improve blood circulation.

Ingredients: Blood purifiers may contain a variety of herbs and botanical extracts known for their purported cleansing and detoxifying properties. Common ingredients include burdock root, red clover, dandelion root, and yellow dock root, among others.

How to Prepare: Blood purifiers are typically available in various forms, including capsules, tablets, powders, and liquid extracts. They are usually taken orally with water or juice, following the recommended dosage on the product label.

Dosage: The dosage of blood purifiers can vary depending on the specific product and individual needs. It's important to adhere to the recommended dosage on the product label or consult with a healthcare professional for personalized guidance.

How to Use: Blood purifiers are typically taken orally, either with water or mixed into beverages. They are often used as part of a detoxification regimen or to support overall health and vitality.

Side Effects: While blood purifiers are generally considered safe for most people when used as directed, some individuals may experience side effects such as digestive discomfort, allergic reactions, or interactions with medications. It's important to consult with a healthcare provider before starting any new supplement regimen, especially if you have underlying health conditions or are taking medications.

Blue Vervain:

Definition: Blue vervain, also known as Verbena hastata, is a perennial herb native to North America. It has been used in traditional medicine for centuries to treat various ailments, including anxiety, insomnia, and digestive issues.

Ingredients: Blue vervain contains several active compounds, including aucubin, verbenalin, and volatile oils. These compounds are believed to contribute to the herb's medicinal properties.

How to Prepare: Blue vervain is typically consumed as a tea or tincture. To make tea, dried blue vervain leaves and flowers are steeped in hot water for several minutes before being strained and consumed. Tinctures are prepared by steeping the herb in alcohol or vinegar to extract its active compounds.

Dosage: The appropriate dosage of blue vervain can vary depending on factors such as age, health status, and the specific preparation being used. It's important to follow the recommended dosage on the product label or consult with a qualified herbalist or healthcare professional for personalized guidance.

How to Use: Blue vervain tea or tincture is typically taken orally. It can be consumed on its own or mixed with honey or other herbal teas for added flavor.

Side Effects: While blue vervain is generally considered safe for most people when used in moderation, excessive intake may cause digestive upset or allergic reactions in some individuals. Pregnant or breastfeeding women should avoid blue vervain due to its potential to stimulate uterine contractions. As with any herbal remedy, it's important to consult with a healthcare provider before using blue vervain, especially if you have underlying health conditions or are taking medications.

Bromide Plus Powder:

Definition: Bromide Plus Powder is a dietary supplement formulated to support thyroid health and promote overall well-being. It typically contains a blend of herbs and minerals that are believed to have beneficial effects on thyroid function.

Ingredients: Bromide Plus Powder often contains a combination of herbs such as bladderwrack, sea moss, and burdock root, along with minerals like iodine and potassium phosphate. These ingredients are thought to support thyroid function and maintain optimal iodine levels in the body.

How to Prepare: Bromide Plus Powder is usually mixed with water or juice to create a drinkable solution. It's important to follow the instructions on the product label for dosage and preparation.

Dosage: The dosage of Bromide Plus Powder can vary depending on the specific product and individual needs. It's crucial to consult with a healthcare professional or follow the recommended dosage on the product label to avoid potential side effects.

How to Use: Bromide Plus Powder is typically taken orally by mixing the recommended dosage with water or juice. It's important to shake or stir the mixture well before consuming it to ensure even distribution of the ingredients.

Side Effects: While Bromide Plus Powder is generally considered safe when used as directed, some individuals may experience side effects such as digestive discomfort or allergic reactions to certain ingredients. It's essential to consult with a healthcare provider before starting any new supplement regimen, especially if you have underlying health conditions or are taking medications.

Bugleweed:

Definition: Bugleweed, also known as Lycopusvirginicus, is a perennial herb native to North America and Europe. It has been used in traditional medicine to treat various conditions, including hyperthyroidism, anxiety, and insomnia.

Ingredients: Bugleweed contains several active compounds, including lithospermic acid, phenolic acids, and flavonoids. These compounds are believed to contribute to the herb's medicinal properties, particularly its ability to regulate thyroid function.

How to Prepare: Bugleweed is commonly consumed as a tea or tincture. To make tea, dried bugleweed leaves and flowers are steeped in hot water for several minutes before being strained and consumed. Tinctures are prepared by steeping the herb in alcohol or vinegar to extract its active compounds.

Dosage: The appropriate dosage of bugleweed can vary depending on factors such as age, health status, and the specific preparation being used. It's important to follow the recommended dosage on the product label or consult with a qualified herbalist or healthcare professional for personalized guidance.

How to Use: Bugleweed tea or tincture is typically taken orally. It can be consumed on its own or mixed with honey or other herbal teas for added flavor.

Side Effects: While bugleweed is generally considered safe for most people when used in moderation, excessive intake may cause digestive upset or allergic reactions in some individuals. Pregnant or breastfeeding women should avoid bugleweed due to its potential to stimulate uterine contractions. As with any herbal remedy, it's important to consult with a healthcare provider before using bugleweed, especially if you have underlying health conditions or are taking medications.

Burdock:

Definition: Burdock, scientifically known as Arctium lappa, is a biennial plant native to Europe and Asia but now found worldwide. It's part of the Asteraceae family and has been used for centuries in traditional medicine and culinary practices.

Ingredients: Burdock contains various nutrients, including carbohydrates, fiber, vitamins (such as vitamin B6, folate, and vitamin C), and minerals (including potassium, magnesium, and manganese). It also contains active compounds such as polyphenols and volatile oils.

How to Prepare: Burdock can be prepared and consumed in various ways. The roots, leaves, and seeds are all utilized for different purposes. The root is commonly used in cooking, herbal teas, tinctures, and supplements, while the leaves and seeds are sometimes used in herbal preparations.

Dosage: The appropriate dosage of burdock root can vary depending on the specific form and intended use. For culinary purposes, there are no strict dosage guidelines, but for supplements or herbal remedies, it's essential to follow the recommended dosage on the product label or consult with a healthcare professional.

How to Use: Burdock root can be used in cooking by peeling, slicing, and adding it to soups, stews, stir-fries, or salads. It can also be brewed into a tea or used to make tinctures or extracts for medicinal purposes. Some people may also take burdock root supplements in capsule or powder form.

Side Effects: While burdock is generally considered safe for most people when consumed in moderate amounts, some individuals may experience allergic reactions or digestive upset. Additionally, burdock may interact with certain medications or have adverse effects in individuals with certain health conditions, such as diabetes or allergies to plants in the Asteraceae family. It's important to consult with a healthcare provider before using burdock, especially if you have underlying health conditions or are taking medications.

Cascara Sagrada:

Definition: Cascara Sagrada, scientifically known as Rhamnus purshiana, is a species of buckthorn native to western North America. It has been used traditionally as a laxative and to promote bowel regularity.

Ingredients: The primary active ingredients in cascara sagrada are anthraquinone glycosides, particularly cascarosides A and B. These compounds stimulate peristalsis in the colon, leading to increased bowel movements.

How to Prepare: Cascara sagrada is typically prepared as an herbal tea, tincture, or capsule. To make tea, dried cascara sagrada bark is steeped in hot water for several minutes before being strained and consumed. Tinctures are prepared by steeping the bark in alcohol to extract its active compounds.

Dosage: The appropriate dosage of cascara sagrada can vary depending on the specific preparation and intended use. It's important to follow the recommended dosage on the product label or consult with a healthcare professional for personalized guidance.

How to Use: Cascara sagrada tea or tincture is typically taken orally. It's important to start with a low dose and gradually increase if needed to avoid potential side effects such as cramping or diarrhea.

Side Effects: Cascara sagrada is considered safe for short-term use when used as directed. However, long-term or excessive use may lead to dependence, electrolyte imbalance, or dehydration. It may also interact with certain medications or have adverse effects in individuals with certain health conditions. It's important to use cascara sagrada under the guidance of a healthcare professional and to discontinue use if any adverse effects occur.

Cell Food:

Definition: Cell Food is a dietary supplement marketed as a highly oxygenating and alkalizing formula. It's claimed to support overall health and vitality by providing essential nutrients and oxygen to the cells.

Ingredients: The exact ingredients of Cell Food can vary depending on the brand, but it typically contains a proprietary blend of minerals, enzymes, electrolytes, and trace elements. Some common ingredients may include purified water, dissolved oxygen, seawater extract, and plant-based enzymes.

How to Prepare: Cell Food is usually available in liquid form and is typically taken orally. It can be consumed directly or diluted in water or juice before consumption.

Dosage: The dosage of Cell Food can vary depending on the specific product and individual needs. It's important to follow the recommended dosage on the product label or consult with a healthcare professional for personalized guidance.

How to Use: Cell Food is typically taken orally, either directly or mixed into water or juice. It's important to shake the bottle well before use and to store it according to the manufacturer's instructions.

Side Effects: Cell Food is generally considered safe for most people when used as directed. However, some individuals may experience mild digestive upset or allergic reactions to certain ingredients. It's essential to consult with a healthcare provider before starting any new supplement regimen, especially if you have underlying health conditions or are taking medications.

Chaparral:

Definition: Chaparral, scientifically known as Larrea tridentata, is a shrub native to the southwestern United States and northern Mexico. It has been used for centuries by Native American tribes for its medicinal properties and is commonly used in herbal medicine today.

Ingredients: Chaparral contains several bioactive compounds, including nordihydroguaiaretic acid (NDGA), flavonoids, lignans, and volatile oils. NDGA is believed to be the primary active compound responsible for many of chaparral's therapeutic effects.

How to Prepare: Chaparral can be prepared and consumed in various forms, including teas, tinctures, capsules, and topical preparations. To make tea, dried chaparral leaves are steeped in hot water for several minutes before being strained and consumed. Tinctures are prepared by steeping the herb in alcohol or vinegar to extract its active compounds.

Dosage: The appropriate dosage of chaparral can vary depending on the specific form and intended use. It's important to follow the recommended dosage on the product label or consult with a healthcare professional for personalized guidance.

How to Use: Chaparral tea or tincture is typically taken orally. It can also be applied topically to the skin for certain conditions. It's important to use chaparral products as directed and to discontinue use if any adverse effects occur.

Side Effects: Chaparral is generally considered safe for most people when used in moderate amounts. However, excessive intake or prolonged use may lead to liver toxicity or other adverse effects. It may also interact with certain medications or have adverse effects in individuals with certain health conditions. It's important to use chaparral under the guidance of a healthcare professional and to discontinue use if any adverse effects occur.

Cocolmeca:

Definition: Cocolmeca, also known as Smilax ornata or sarsaparilla, is a flowering vine native to Mexico and Central America. It has been used traditionally in Mexican and Central American folk medicine for its purported medicinal properties.

Ingredients: Cocolmeca contains various bioactive compounds, including saponins, flavonoids, and plant sterols. These compounds are believed to contribute to the herb's medicinal properties, including its potential as a diuretic, blood purifier, and anti-inflammatory agent.

How to Prepare: Cocolmeca is commonly prepared and consumed as an herbal tea or decoction. To make tea, dried cocolmeca roots or leaves are steeped in hot water for several minutes before being strained and consumed. Decoctions involve boiling the roots or leaves in water to extract their active compounds.

Dosage: The appropriate dosage of cocolmeca can vary depending on factors such as age, health status, and the specific preparation being used. It's important to follow the recommended dosage on the product label or consult with a qualified herbalist or healthcare professional for personalized guidance.

How to Use: Cocolmeca tea or decoction is typically taken orally. It can also be used topically for certain skin conditions. It's important to use cocolmeca products as directed and to discontinue use if any adverse effects occur.

Side Effects: Cocolmeca is generally considered safe for most people when used in moderate amounts. However, excessive intake may lead to digestive upset or other adverse effects. It may also interact with certain medications or have adverse effects in individuals with certain health conditions. It's important to use cocolmeca under the guidance of a healthcare professional and to discontinue use if any adverse effects occur.

Contribo:

Definition: Contribo, also known as Aristolochiatrilobata, is a vine native to the Caribbean and Central America. It has been used traditionally in folk medicine for various purposes, including as a remedy for digestive issues, inflammation, and pain relief.

Ingredients: Contribo contains several bioactive compounds, including aristolochic acids, flavonoids, and alkaloids. These compounds are believed to contribute to the herb's medicinal properties, including its potential as an anti-inflammatory and analgesic agent.

How to Prepare: Contribo is typically prepared and consumed as an herbal tea or decoction. To make tea, dried contribo leaves or stems are steeped in hot water for several minutes before being strained and consumed. Decoctions involve boiling the leaves or stems in water to extract their active compounds.

Dosage: The appropriate dosage of contribo can vary depending on factors such as age, health status, and the specific preparation being used. It's important to follow the recommended dosage on the product label or consult with a qualified herbalist or healthcare professional for personalized guidance.

How to Use: Contribo tea or decoction is typically taken orally. It's important to use contribo products as directed and to discontinue use if any adverse effects occur.

Side Effects: Contribo contains aristolochic acids, which have been associated with serious adverse effects, including kidney damage and cancer. Due to these safety concerns, the use of contribo is highly discouraged, and it's important to avoid products containing aristolochic acids. Individuals should seek alternative remedies for their health needs.

Dandelion Root:

Definition: Dandelion, scientifically known as Taraxacum officinale, is a common flowering plant found worldwide. While often considered a pesky weed, dandelion has a long history of use in traditional medicine for its various health benefits.

Ingredients: Dandelion root contains several bioactive compounds, including sesquiterpene lactones, triterpenes, flavonoids, and polysaccharides. These compounds are believed to contribute to the herb's medicinal properties, including its potential as a diuretic, digestive aid, and liver tonic.

How to Prepare: Dandelion root can be prepared and consumed in various forms, including teas, tinctures, capsules, and extracts. To make tea, dried dandelion root is steeped in hot water for several minutes before being strained and consumed. Tinctures are prepared by steeping the root in alcohol or vinegar to extract its active compounds.

Dosage: The appropriate dosage of dandelion root can vary depending on factors such as age, health status, and the specific preparation being used. It's important to follow the recommended dosage on the product label or consult with a qualified herbalist or healthcare professional for personalized guidance.

How to Use: Dandelion root tea, tincture, or capsules are typically taken orally. It's important to use dandelion root products as directed and to discontinue use if any adverse effects occur.

Side Effects: Dandelion root is generally considered safe for most people when used in moderate amounts. However, some individuals may experience allergic reactions or digestive upset. It may also interact with certain medications or have adverse effects in individuals with certain health conditions. It's important to use dandelion root under the guidance of a healthcare professional and to discontinue use if any adverse effects occur.

Herban Iron:

Definition: Herban Iron is a dietary supplement designed to provide an easily absorbable form of iron to support healthy iron levels in the body. It's particularly beneficial for individuals with iron deficiency or anemia.

Ingredients: Herban Iron typically contains iron in the form of ferrous bisglycinate, which is a highly bioavailable and gentle form of iron that is less likely to cause digestive upset or constipation compared to other forms of iron. It may also contain other ingredients such as vitamin C to enhance iron absorption.

How to Prepare: Herban Iron is usually available in capsule or liquid form. Capsules are taken orally with water, while liquid forms may be mixed with water or juice before consumption. It's important to follow the recommended dosage on the product label.

Dosage: The appropriate dosage of Herban Iron depends on factors such as age, gender, and the severity of iron deficiency. It's important to consult with a healthcare professional to determine the correct dosage for individual needs.

How to Use: Herban Iron capsules are typically taken orally with water, while liquid forms may be mixed with water or juice before consumption. It's important to take Herban Iron as directed and to avoid taking it with dairy products, antacids, or other substances that may interfere with iron absorption.

Side Effects: While Herban Iron is generally considered safe for most people when used as directed, some individuals may experience mild side effects such as gastrointestinal discomfort or constipation. It's important to consult with a healthcare professional before starting any new supplement regimen, especially if you have underlying health conditions or are taking medications.

Hydrangea:

Definition: Hydrangea, scientifically known as Hydrangea arborescens, is a flowering shrub native to North America. It has been used traditionally in herbal medicine for its potential diuretic and anti-inflammatory properties.

Ingredients: Hydrangea contains several bioactive compounds, including saponins, flavonoids, and glycosides. These compounds are believed to contribute to the herb's medicinal properties, including its potential as a diuretic, kidney tonic, and anti-inflammatory agent.

How to Prepare: Hydrangea root is typically prepared and consumed as an herbal tea or tincture. To make tea, dried hydrangea root is steeped in hot water for several minutes before being strained and consumed. Tinctures are prepared by steeping the root in alcohol or vinegar to extract its active compounds.

Dosage: The appropriate dosage of hydrangea can vary depending on factors such as age, health status, and the specific preparation being used. It's important to follow the recommended dosage on the product label or consult with a qualified herbalist or healthcare professional for personalized guidance.

How to Use: Hydrangea tea or tincture is typically taken orally. It's important to use hydrangea products as directed and to discontinue use if any adverse effects occur.

Side Effects: Hydrangea is generally considered safe for most people when used in moderate amounts. However, some individuals may experience digestive upset or allergic reactions. It may also interact with certain medications or have adverse effects in individuals with certain health conditions. It's important to use hydrangea under the guidance of a healthcare professional and to discontinue use if any adverse effects occur.

Irish Moss:

Definition: Irish Moss, scientifically known as Chondrus crispus, is a species of red algae or seaweed native to the Atlantic coastlines of Europe and North America. It has been used for centuries in traditional Irish and Scottish cuisine, as well as in herbal medicine.

Ingredients: Irish Moss is rich in various nutrients, including iodine, sulfur compounds, vitamins (such as vitamin A, vitamin K, and vitamin B12), minerals (including calcium, magnesium, potassium, and sodium), and polysaccharides (such as carrageenan). These nutrients are believed to contribute to the herb's potential health benefits.

How to Prepare: Irish Moss is typically prepared by soaking it in water to rehydrate and soften it before use. It can be added to soups, stews, smoothies, desserts, and other dishes as a thickening agent or nutritional supplement.

Dosage: The appropriate dosage of Irish Moss can vary depending on factors such as age, health status, and the specific preparation being used. It's important to follow recipes or guidelines for culinary use and to consult with a healthcare professional for guidance on using Irish Moss as a dietary supplement.

How to Use: Irish Moss can be used in culinary applications to add thickness and nutritional value to dishes. It can also be consumed as a dietary supplement in the form of capsules, powders, or extracts.

Side Effects: Irish Moss is generally considered safe for most people when consumed in moderate amounts as part of a balanced diet. However, some individuals may be allergic to seaweed or carrageenan, a compound found in Irish Moss that is used as a food additive. It's important to discontinue use if any adverse effects occur and to consult with a healthcare professional if you have any concerns.

Irish Sea Moss:

Definition: Irish Sea Moss is a term often used interchangeably with Irish Moss, referring to the same species of red algae, Chondrus crispus. It's harvested from the rocky shores of the Atlantic coastlines of Europe and North America.

Ingredients: Irish Sea Moss shares the same nutritional profile as Irish Moss, containing iodine, vitamins, minerals, and polysaccharides. It's valued for its potential health benefits, including supporting thyroid function, boosting immune health, and promoting digestion.

How to Prepare: Irish Sea Moss is prepared in the same way as Irish Moss, by soaking it in water to rehydrate and soften it before use. It can be used in culinary applications or consumed as a dietary supplement.

Dosage: The dosage of Irish Sea Moss depends on the form and intended use. As a dietary supplement, it's important to follow the recommended dosage on the product label or consult with a healthcare professional for personalized guidance.

How to Use: Irish Sea Moss can be used in various culinary applications, including soups, smoothies, desserts, and sauces. It can also be consumed as a dietary supplement in the form of capsules, powders, or extracts.

Side Effects: Similar to Irish Moss, Irish Sea Moss is generally considered safe for most people when consumed in moderate amounts. However, individuals with seaweed allergies or sensitivities to carrageenan should exercise caution. It's important to discontinue use if any adverse effects occur and to consult with a healthcare professional if you have any concerns.

Lymphalin:

Definition: Lymphalin is a herbal supplement formulated to support lymphatic system health. The lymphatic system plays a crucial role in immune function and waste removal in the body, and Lymphalin is designed to promote its proper function.

Ingredients: Lymphalin typically contains a blend of herbs and botanical extracts known for their traditional use in supporting lymphatic system health. Common ingredients may include cleavers, red clover, echinacea, burdock root, and calendula, among others.

How to Prepare: Lymphalin is usually available in capsule or liquid form. Capsules are taken orally with water, while liquid forms may be mixed with water or juice before consumption. It's important to follow the recommended dosage on the product label.

Dosage: The appropriate dosage of Lymphalin can vary depending on the specific product and individual needs. It's important to follow the recommended dosage on the product label or consult with a healthcare professional for personalized guidance.

How to Use: Lymphalin capsules are typically taken orally with water, while liquid forms may be mixed with water or juice before consumption. It's often recommended to take Lymphalin on an empty stomach for optimal absorption.

Side Effects: Lymphalin is generally considered safe for most people when used as directed. However, some individuals may experience mild side effects such as gastrointestinal discomfort or allergic reactions to certain ingredients. It's important to consult with a healthcare provider before starting any new supplement regimen, especially if you have underlying health conditions or are taking medications.

Manjakani:

Definition: Manjakani, also known as Quercus infectoria or oak gall, is a natural substance derived from the oak tree. It has been used for centuries in traditional medicine for its potential health benefits, particularly for women's health and vaginal tightening.

Ingredients: Manjakani contains various bioactive compounds, including tannins, flavonoids, and gallic acid. These compounds are believed to contribute to the herb's medicinal properties, including its potential as an astringent and antiseptic agent.

How to Prepare: Manjakani is typically available in powder, capsule, or liquid extract form. It can be taken orally or used topically depending on the intended use. For vaginal tightening, manjakani may be applied topically as a gel or inserted into the vagina in capsule form.

Dosage: The appropriate dosage of manjakani can vary depending on factors such as age, health status, and the specific preparation being used. It's important to follow the recommended dosage on the product label or consult with a qualified herbalist or healthcare professional for personalized guidance.

How to Use: Manjakani can be taken orally or used topically depending on the intended use. It's important to use manjakani products as directed and to discontinue use if any adverse effects occur.

Side Effects: Manjakani is generally considered safe for most people when used in moderate amounts. However, some individuals may experience allergic reactions or skin irritation when used topically. It's important to use manjakani under the guidance of a healthcare professional and to discontinue use if any adverse effects occur.

Red Clover:

Definition: Red clover, scientifically known as Trifolium pratense, is a flowering plant belonging to the legume family. It's native to Europe, Western Asia, and Northwest Africa but has been naturalized in many other regions. Red clover has been used in traditional medicine for various purposes, including its potential to support women's health and menopausal symptoms.

Ingredients: Red clover contains several bioactive compounds, including isoflavones (such as genistein and daidzein), flavonoids, and phytoestrogens. These compounds are believed to contribute to the herb's medicinal properties, including its potential as a hormone-balancing agent and its ability to support cardiovascular health.

How to Prepare: Red clover is typically prepared and consumed as an herbal tea or tincture. To make tea, dried red clover flowers are steeped in hot water for several minutes before being strained and consumed. Tinctures are prepared by steeping the flowers in alcohol or vinegar to extract their active compounds.

Dosage: The appropriate dosage of red clover can vary depending on factors such as age, health status, and the specific preparation being used. It's important to follow the recommended dosage on the product label or consult with a qualified herbalist or healthcare professional for personalized guidance.

How to Use: Red clover tea or tincture is typically taken orally. It's important to use red clover products as directed and to discontinue use if any adverse effects occur.

Side Effects: Red clover is generally considered safe for most people when used in moderate amounts. However, some individuals may experience allergic reactions or digestive upset. It may also interact with certain medications or have adverse effects in individuals with certain health conditions. It's important to use red clover under the guidance of a healthcare professional and to discontinue use if any adverse effects occur.

Red Raspberry:

Definition: Red raspberry, scientifically known as Rubus idaeus, is a species of raspberry native to Europe and northern Asia. It's widely cultivated for its delicious berries and has been used in traditional medicine for various purposes, including its potential to support women's health during pregnancy and childbirth.

Ingredients: Red raspberry contains several bioactive compounds, including flavonoids, ellagic acid, anthocyanins, and vitamin C. These compounds are believed to contribute to the herb's medicinal properties, including its potential as an antioxidant, anti-inflammatory, and uterine tonic.

How to Prepare: Red raspberry leaf is typically prepared and consumed as an herbal tea or infusion. To make tea, dried red raspberry leaves are steeped in hot water for several minutes before being strained and consumed.

Dosage: The appropriate dosage of red raspberry leaf can vary depending on factors such as age, health status, and the specific preparation being used. It's important to follow the recommended dosage on the product label or consult with a qualified herbalist or healthcare professional for personalized guidance.

How to Use: Red raspberry leaf tea is typically taken orally. It's often recommended for pregnant individuals in the later stages of pregnancy to support uterine health and prepare for childbirth. It's important to use red raspberry leaf products as directed and to discontinue use if any adverse effects occur.

Side Effects: Red raspberry leaf is generally considered safe for most people when used in moderate amounts. However, some individuals may experience allergic reactions or digestive upset. Pregnant individuals should consult with a healthcare professional before using red raspberry leaf, especially if they have any underlying health conditions or are taking medications. It's important to use red raspberry leaf under the guidance of a healthcare professional and to discontinue use if any adverse effects occur.

Rhubarb:

Definition: Rhubarb, scientifically known as Rheum rhabarbarum, is a perennial plant cultivated for its edible stalks. While primarily used in culinary applications, rhubarb has also been utilized in traditional medicine for its potential health benefits, particularly for digestive health.

Ingredients: Rhubarb stalks contain various bioactive compounds, including anthraquinones (such as emodin and rhein), fiber, vitamins (such as vitamin K), and minerals (including calcium and potassium). These compounds are believed to contribute to the herb's medicinal properties, including its potential as a laxative and digestive aid.

How to Prepare: Rhubarb stalks are typically cooked before consumption, as the raw stalks are very tart and can be unpleasant to eat. They are often used in pies, crisps, jams, sauces, and other desserts, as well as in savory dishes. Rhubarb can also be used to make compotes, jams, and preserves.

Dosage: There is no specific dosage for rhubarb in culinary applications, as it is used as a food rather than a medicinal herb. However, when used for its potential laxative effects, it's important to consume rhubarb in moderation to avoid gastrointestinal upset.

How to Use: Rhubarb stalks can be chopped and cooked in various dishes, including pies, sauces, and jams. It's important to remove and discard the leaves, as they contain toxic compounds.

When using rhubarb for its potential laxative effects, it's typically consumed as part of a cooked dish or in the form of a rhubarb-based herbal remedy.

Side Effects: Rhubarb stalks are generally safe for most people when consumed in moderate amounts as part of a balanced diet. However, excessive intake may lead to digestive upset or adverse effects due to the presence of oxalic acid, which can bind to calcium and form kidney stones in susceptible individuals. It's important to use rhubarb in moderation and to consult with a healthcare professional if you have any concerns or underlying health conditions.

Guaco:

Definition: Guaco, also known as Mikania cordata or Mikania glomerata, is a medicinal plant native to Central and South America. It has a long history of use in traditional medicine for its potential therapeutic properties.

Ingredients: Guaco contains several bioactive compounds, including coumarins, flavonoids, tannins, and saponins. These compounds are believed to contribute to the herb's medicinal properties, including its potential as an expectorant, anti-inflammatory, and antispasmodic agent.

How to Prepare: Guaco is typically prepared and consumed as an herbal tea or infusion. To make tea, dried guaco leaves are steeped in hot water for several minutes before being strained and consumed.

Dosage: The appropriate dosage of guaco can vary depending on factors such as age, health status, and the specific preparation being used. It's important to follow the recommended dosage on the product label or consult with a qualified herbalist or healthcare professional for personalized guidance.

How to Use: Guaco tea is typically taken orally. It can be consumed on its own or mixed with honey or other herbal teas for added flavor.

Side Effects: Guaco is generally considered safe for most people when used in moderate amounts. However, some individuals may experience allergic reactions or digestive upset. It may also interact with certain medications or have adverse effects in individuals with certain health conditions. It's important to use guaco under the guidance of a healthcare professional and to discontinue use if any adverse effects occur.

Hops:

Definition: Hops, scientifically known as Humulus lupulus, is a perennial climbing vine native to Europe, Asia, and North America. It is primarily known for its use in brewing beer but has also been used historically in traditional medicine for its potential health benefits.

Ingredients: Hops flowers contain various bioactive compounds, including bitter acids (such as humulone and lupulone), essential oils, flavonoids, and polyphenols. These compounds are believed to contribute to the herb's medicinal properties, including its potential as a sedative, relaxant, and digestive aid.

How to Prepare: Hops is typically consumed as an herbal tea, tincture, or in supplement form (such as capsules or tablets). To make tea, dried hops flowers are steeped in hot water for several minutes before being strained and consumed.

Dosage: The appropriate dosage of hops can vary depending on factors such as age, health status, and the specific preparation being used. It's important to follow the recommended dosage on the product label or consult with a qualified herbalist or healthcare professional for personalized guidance.

How to Use: Hops tea, tincture, or supplements are typically taken orally. It's often used to promote relaxation, relieve anxiety, and support sleep.

Side Effects: Hops is generally considered safe for most people when used in moderate amounts. However, some individuals may experience mild side effects such as drowsiness, gastrointestinal upset, or allergic reactions. It may also interact with certain medications or have adverse effects in individuals with certain health conditions, such as depression or hormone-sensitive conditions. It's important to use hops under the guidance of a healthcare professional and to discontinue use if any adverse effects occur.

Kelp:

Definition: Kelp refers to several species of large brown algae belonging to the Laminariales order. It is commonly found in underwater forests along rocky coastlines around the world. Kelp has been used for centuries in various cultures, particularly in East Asia, for its nutritional and medicinal properties.

Ingredients: Kelp is rich in various nutrients, including iodine, vitamins (such as vitamin K, vitamin C, and B vitamins), minerals (including calcium, magnesium, and potassium), antioxidants, and fiber. These nutrients are believed to contribute to the seaweed's potential health benefits, including its role in thyroid function, bone health, and immune support.

How to Prepare: Kelp is typically consumed dried, powdered, or in supplement form (such as capsules or tablets). It can also be used in cooking, particularly in soups, salads, and stir-fries. Kelp supplements are available in various forms, including powdered extracts, tablets, and liquid extracts.

Dosage: The appropriate dosage of kelp can vary depending on factors such as age, health status, and the specific preparation being used. It's important to follow the recommended dosage on the product label or consult with a qualified healthcare professional for personalized guidance.

How to Use: Kelp supplements are typically taken orally with water. They can be consumed as part of a daily nutritional regimen to support overall health and well-being. Kelp can also be incorporated into recipes as a flavorful and nutritious ingredient.

Side Effects: While kelp is generally considered safe for most people when consumed in moderate amounts, excessive intake of iodine-rich foods or supplements, including kelp, can lead to thyroid dysfunction or iodine toxicity. Some individuals may also be allergic to seaweed and experience allergic reactions. Pregnant or breastfeeding individuals should consult with a healthcare professional before using kelp supplements. It's important to use kelp under the guidance of a healthcare professional and to discontinue use if any adverse effects occur.

THE END

www.ingramcontent.com/pod-product-compliance
Lightning Source LLC
Chambersburg PA
CBHW081558250726
48653CB00009B/3488